Handbook for Newly Diagnosed Cases of Adhesive Arachnoiditis

A Ten-Step Plan to Relief and Recovery

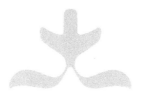

Forest Tennant
(DrPH, MPH, MD)

Published by the
Tennant Foundation
West Covina, California

Copyright© 2023 Tennant Foundation

All rights reserved. This book or any portion thereof may not be reproduced or used in any manner whatsoever without the express written permission of the publisher except for the use of brief quotations in a book review or scholarly journal.

ISBN: 9781955934244
Library of Congress Control Number: 2023908116

Special discounts are available on quantity purchases by corporations, associations, educators, and others. For details, contact one of the parties listed below.

U.S. trade bookstores and wholesalers: Please contact
Nancy Kriskovich Tel: (406)249-2002;
or email snkriskovich@gmail.com

All proceeds from the sale of this book will go to the Medical Study and Education Projects sponsored by the
Tennant Foundation
336-338 S. Glendora Ave.
West Covina, CA 91790-3043
Ph: 626-716-2689
Fax: 626-919-7497
Email: tennantfoundation92@gmail.com

BOARD OF DIRECTORS
Chairperson: Jerry Muszynski
President: Forest Tennant
Vice President: Miriam Tennant
Secretary: Kathy Clark
Treasurer: James Hetzel

BOARD MEMBERS
Doran Barnes
Steve Castillo
Sander De Wildt
Brad Manning
Don Scheliga
Vicki Scheliga
Tony Song
Ken Yoho

STUDY AND EDUCATION COMMITTEE

Terri Anderson
Lynn Ashcraft
Andy Boyles
Donna Corley
Mark Ibsen, MD
K. Scott Guess, Pharm D
Ryle Holder, Pharm D
Nancy Kriskovich
Kristen Ogden
Rhonda Posey
Jaime Sanchez, RN
Gary Snook

MEDICAL DIRECTOR
Martin J. Porcelli, DO, MHPE, PhD

ACKNOWLEDGEMENTS
This book could not have been researched and written without the technical assistance of Becky and Tom Marino, Nancy Kriskovich, and Jaime Sanchez, RN.

DEDICATION

This handbook is dedicated to Rhonda Posey, for her tireless efforts in developing self-help measures for persons with adhesive arachnoiditis.

Table of Contents

Author's Message to New Cases of Adhesive Arachnoiditis...1

Introduction 4

The Disease of AA 6

Medical Treatment Protocol 9

Some Do's and Don'ts 10

First Goal: Stop Deterioration..............................12

Step One: Begin Nutritional Measures and Diet.....13

Step Two: Embark on Key Physical Measures 15

Step Three: Continue Measures That Work...........17

Step Four: Start Topical Treatment 18

Step Five: Assess What Matters Most...................20

Step Six: Pull Out Retained Electricity 22

Step Seven: Determine Your Causes and Stage of AA..25

Step Eight: Start Treatment with Natural and Herbal Agents..28

Step Nine: Prepare to Seek Medical Help 31

Step Ten: Start Spinal Fluid Flow Exercises..........34

Summary..37

Appendix 39

- A. Symptom Criteria for the Diagnosis of AA .39
- B. Consequences and Complications of AA 40
- C. Stages and Categorizations of AA 43
- D. Diagnostic Screening Test for Ehlers Danlos Syndromes (EDS)..45
- E. Diagnostic Screening Test for An Autoimmune Disorder 47
- F. Start and Stop Rule for Pharmaceuticals.....49
- G. Physician's Starting Three Component Medical Protocol..51

Glossary of Terms 54

References 57

Index..62

Author's Message to New Cases of Adhesive Arachnoiditis

When one first receives a diagnosis of adhesive arachnoiditis (AA), it is natural to feel frightened, depressed, and hopeless. This handbook is to help you get over these feelings and develop a treatment program for relief and recovery. Many years ago, it was often called the "Devil's Disease." No wonder. There was no treatment and most persons afflicted with it died within a year or two after their initial diagnosis.

Today, it is a totally different situation. Treatment isn't a single drug, and AA may not be curable, but it is now very treatable. Practically every person with AA can achieve at least some relief and recovery. Near cure is even possible with an early diagnosis and aggressive treatment. A high-quality long lifespan is now the rule rather than the exception. In summary,

Handbook for Newly Diagnosed Cases of AA

don't let any physician or anyone else tell you that there is no treatment or "nothing can be done."

This handbook has ten steps to get you started. You will need a physician's help to prescribe some drugs. Most of the treatment, however, is strictly something you can and must do for yourself to prevent AA from becoming progressively worse.

There is a set of nutritional and physical measures that are essential to control pain and prevent neurologic impairments. You should start some of them today.

This handbook is not a guide for treatment after sixty days. At that time, you and your medical care practitioners will want to pick and choose among multiple choices you have to enhance the treatment program you initiated.

Forest Tennant (DrPH, MPH, MD)

*This handbook only refers to lumbar-sacral adhesive arachnoiditis unless specifically noted.

**Physician includes medical practitioners licensed to prescribe including nurse practitioners, physician's assistants, and naturopaths.

Introduction

Adhesive arachnoiditis (AA) is a most serious inflammatory-autoimmune disease in which some cauda equina nerve roots are adhered by adhesions to the arachnoid layer of the spinal canal covering (meninges). In the past, the major causes have been tuberculosis, syphilis, or toxic dyes that were injected into the spinal canal for x-ray (myelogram) purposes. Today, AA is mostly caused by an autoimmune disorder coupled with a genetic anatomical defect, connective tissue disorder, or traumatic event such as an accident, epidural injection, spinal tap, or surgery. AA has, in the past, been considered a rare disease, but today it is being diagnosed with regularity in every community. It now ranks number one or two among causes of severe intractable pain.

In addition to background information this handbook lays out ten steps to start and build a basic therapeutic program over sixty days. After this time, you will likely want to embark on some specific laboratory testing and additional therapeutics.

The Disease of AA

AA is an inflammatory adhesive mass inside the spinal canal that entraps cauda equina nerve roots. On magnetic resonance imaging (MRI) the mass appears as a clump or group of nerve roots that are stuck together and adhered to the inner lining (i.e., arachnoid membrane) of the spinal canal cover. When cauda equina nerve roots become inflamed and glued to each other and/or to the arachnoid lining of the spinal canal, severe pain and neurologic impairments develop. Since the location of the adhesive clump or mass is in the lumbar-sacral section of the spinal canal, a set of typical symptoms and impairments develop since cauda equina nerve roots have specific neurologic connections and functions. Common symptoms and impairments in addition to severe pain include bladder, sex, and bowel dysfunction, weakened legs, burning feet, restless legs or jerks, and bizarre skin sensations such as insects crawling or water dripping on the legs. A seminal symptom is that pain is relieved by either standing or reclining.

Diagram of Entrapped Nerve Roots in AA

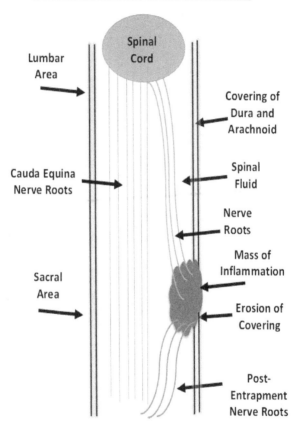

The electricity normally conducted by the cauda equina nerve roots is trapped in the adhesive arachnoid mass and causes pain and inflammation.

Medical Treatment Protocol

A three-component medical protocol is used to treat AA. The medical protocol has three components:

1. Suppression of inflammation and autoimmunity.
2. Regeneration of tissues.
3. Control of pain.

Some specific nutrition and physical measures are necessary to maximize medical treatment. A starting medical protocol for physicians is provided in the Appendix. One of the Steps (No. 8) consists of non-prescription, natural, and herbal agents that a newly diagnosed person can start taking to help prevent disease progression and, ideally, reverse some symptoms.

Some Do's and Don'ts

Here are some simple points to help you focus and get started.

- ➢ Do not panic or become depressed. AA is usually controllable.

- ➢ Do not look for a physician or institution that specializes in AA. They don't yet exist. AA has, until lately, been too rare of a disease for physicians to become knowledgeable about it.

- ➢ Do start reading and educating yourself about AA.

- ➢ Do not rely on a pain clinic since they usually provide only symptomatic pain relief drugs or risky invasive procedures. They don't focus on medication for suppression of inflammation and autoimmunity or to regenerate tissue.

- Do start some of the nutrition and physical measures listed in this handbook. Don't delay because AA can deteriorate and cripple you within a few days or weeks.

- Do join one or more support groups on social media, or in your community.

Do share your concerns and treatment efforts with a close family member or friend.

First Goal: Stop Deterioration

Unfortunately, AA can be a rapid and progressive inflammatory-autoimmune disease that destroys cauda equina nerve root connections to the foot, legs, stomach, intestine, and sex organs. The worst of all pain may ensue. Untreated AA is well-known to cause crippling, paralysis, a bed-bound-sexless life, incontinence, and a shortened lifespan.

Don't delay treatment measures or set some unrealistic goal. Your first concern is simply to keep from getting worse. Don't kill time looking for a medical specialist or some experimental, expensive treatment. Use the ten steps in this handbook to immediately start building your therapy program to stop further deterioration. Once you get started, you and your medical practitioners can make corrections and upgrade your program.

Step One: Begin Nutritional Measures and Diet

Some specific nutritional measures and diet help build a foundation for AA treatment and control. The measures and diet listed here help suppress inflammation and autoimmunity (including viral autoimmunity), regenerate tissue, and control pain.

<u>Daily Measures</u>

A. Vitamins: C (2000 to 4000 mg a day) and B_{12}.
B. Daily minerals: selenium, magnesium, Optional: boron, zinc.
C. Collagen or amino acid supplement.

Diet

a. Eat one or more of these protein foods each meal: beef, lamb, pork, poultry (chicken, turkey), seafood (shrimp, fish, crab), cottage cheese, eggs.
b. Stop drinks that contain sugar (carbohydrates) including fruit juices and soft drinks. Milk is acceptable if you don't gain weight with it.
c. Restrict sugars and starches (e.g., breads, candy, pastries, pasta).
d. Fruits and vegetables of your choice. Green vegetables such as broccoli and beans and some fruits like blueberries and watermelon may reduce inflammation.

Step Two: Embark on Key Physical Measures

Some specific, simple physical measures are critical to prevent deterioration and enhance the effectiveness of medical treatment. Although we recommend all the measures below, select the ones that you will routinely do.

A. Stand and raise your arms straight up to their full extension. Hold for five seconds. Repeat at least six times a day.

B. Stand and support yourself against a wall or tabletop. Keep one leg straight and raise it while you stand on the other. Flex your ankle. Do each leg at least six times a day.

C. Stand straight up and support yourself against a wall or tabletop. Raise one knee and then shift to the other leg. Do each leg at least six times a day.

D. Walk in a straight line and swing your arms for thirty steps at least four times a day. A long walk will substitute.

E. Obtain one-to-three-pound weights and raise them straight up over your head with each arm, three to six times a day.

Step Three: Continue Measures That Work

Chances are you have probably suffered illness for some time and now take a variety of medications and nutritional supplements. Do an inventory of your current medications including dietary supplements and non-prescription aids. Include topical rubs, patches, and devices such as TENS or infrared. Your initial task is to simply identify the ones that "work" to help relieve pain and other symptoms such as insomnia, bladder dysfunction, or fatigue. Keep taking and using what works. You should build your treatment program around drugs and other measures that already work for you.

Step Four: Start Topical Treatment

Topical means "apply to the skin." As a new person with AA, you need to identify some topical treatments that help relieve your pain. Almost all persons with AA have some seepage or leakage of spinal fluid that creeps into the tissues between the spine and skin. AA is an inflammatory disease that erodes through not only the inner arachnoid layer but also the outer dural layer of the spinal canal cover. Spinal fluid that comes in contact with tissues outside the spinal canal causes painful irritation and damage.

Here are some simple measures we recommend:

1. Obtain lidocaine and/or Salonpas™ patches from a local drug store. Apply one to see if you get relief. If so, use as often as needed.

2. Obtain one or more pain relief gels or creams. Some popular ones are arnica, hydrocortisone, aloe vera, and lidocaine. Apply any of these topical creams/gels under a heating pad, hot towel, vibrator, or infrared device.

Don't hesitate to try some other topical or rub-on medications that are not listed here. Just remember that topicals do better when massaged into the skin and/or applied under heat. If and when a topical measure stops working, it often means you have healed the spinal canal covering so that there is no more spinal fluid seepage or leakage.

Step Five: Assess What Matters Most

When you first get the diagnosis of AA, you will probably be a bit "shellshocked." Your mind and thought process may temporarily go "haywire" and illogical. This is a natural reaction. Take heart!! AA isn't going to ruin your life as it has for so many others in the past when there was no treatment. You may have to make a few adjustments, but you can now lead a good quality, long life with AA.

Sit down by yourself and take an inventory of what really matters in your life and what gives you joy. What gives you the will to carry on? Who's important in your life? Who is your God and what spiritual journey have you taken?

Knowing what really counts in your life makes it much easier and meaningful to set treatment goals. It may also make it easier to take some risks or even try some experimental treatments.

If possible, share what matters most with your loved ones or close friends.

You may be surprised at "what matters most." Once you truly know "what matters" you can build your therapeutic program to make sure you stay on track with your inner self.

Step Six: Pull Out Retained Electricity

AA entraps nerve roots so electricity normally generated in them cannot travel up and down the nerve roots as usual. If there is nerve root damage, electricity will back-up and accumulate to be later released in an abnormal way. Usually, it is in spurts or too much at one time. This physiologic process is believed to be responsible not only for heat, sweating, and increased temperature and pain, but the cause of abnormal skin sensations (bugs or water dripping), jerks, restless legs, and burning feet. Retention of electricity is believed by many medical experts to be a cause of small nerve fiber neuropathies. If you have AA, you will need to do some daily measures to reduce retained electricity. Here are some simple measures you can start today.

1. Water Soaking-Daily

Water pulls out retained electricity. Warm water is best. Minerals such as Epsom Salts help. Ideally a daily soak in a pool or jacuzzi is optimal. Few people, however, have access to either. Use a bathtub to soak if you are physically able to get in and out of a tub.

Alternatively, take a shower and run warm water over your back. Foot soaking with Epsom or herbal salts in the water may be helpful.

2. Magnet

Magnet rubs over your back or the placement of a magnet in your shoes or under your mattress may be helpful. Magnets force retained electricity to move. If magnet therapy works for you, it will be obvious as pain will reduce, and your body will be more flexible.

3. <u>Copper</u>

Copper and metal jewelry attract electricity. You can rub a piece of copper over your back and spine, and/or wear a copper bracelet or anklet. As with magnet therapy, you will know if copper is helping. Pain will reduce and you will experience enhanced body flexibility.

4. <u>Fur Rubs</u>

Rubbing fur may pull out some retained electricity. In other words, see that your cat or dog gets lots of petting!!

In summary, electricity produced in entrapped or damaged cauda equina nerve roots may accumulate or "back up." Retained electricity may worsen inflammation, pain, and most importantly, increase the risk that AA may deteriorate. The remedies listed here aren't classified as "highly scientific" or "evidence-based", but they have been around for centuries, and most persons with AA claim some benefit from them.

Step Seven: Determine Your Causes and Stage of AA

In years gone by AA was almost always resulted from a single cause such as tuberculosis or dye used for myelograms. Today AA is almost always caused by a combination of two or more factors. A person with AA will have to inform various parties within the health system as to why they have such a serious disease. This will include physicians, pharmacies, and health insurance carriers.

The basic factor that leads to AA is some anatomic abnormality of the spinal cord tissues. This abnormality can be a genetic defect such as scoliosis or a connective tissue disorder called Ehlers-Danlos Syndrome. Trauma due to an accident or a medical procedure such as an epidural injection can also cause an anatomic defect to occur. Medical procedures or traumatic accidents may permit a toxic substance to enter the spinal canal. The second factor is an autoimmune disorder that can be either acquired or genetic. Autoimmune is simply defined as a destructive element in your body that is eating away and eroding the collagen in your tissues causing severe pain and physiologic impairments. The destructive element can be a chemical, toxin, enzyme, germ, or antibody. In the Appendix there is a diagnostic screening test that will give you an idea whether you have an autoimmune disorder.

Anatomic Defects in Spinal Cord Tissues

Trauma*
1. Accident
2. Epidural injection
3. Spine surgery
4. Spinal tap

Genetic
1. Rheumatoid spondylitis
2. Ehlers-Danlos Syndromes (connective tissue)
3. Scoliosis
5. Spondylolisthesis

Autoimmune Disorders

Genetic
1. Systemic lupus erythematosus (SLE)
2. Rheumatoid arthritis
3. Psoriasis

Infection
1. Viral (Epstein Barr, cytomegalovirus)
2. Lyme disease

*Trauma to spinal cord tissues may allow or cause some toxic material to enter the spinal canal.

Not only will you need to know the causes of your AA, you will need to know which stage you are in. AA has four categories: (1) mild, (2) moderate, (3) severe, and (4) catastrophic. Review the classification in the Appendix. If you are in the mild or moderate category, you need to put focus on suppression of inflammation and autoimmunity. If you are in the severe or catastrophic categories, you need to put your focus on regeneration of tissue and pain control.

Step Eight: Start Treatment with Natural and Herbal Agents

To get started with treatment, obtain the following non-prescription, medicinal agents shown in the Table. All are herbal or natural (made in the human body) medicinal agents. The physician's starting three component medical protocol is in the Appendix. While searching or waiting for physician care, get started with the herbal and natural agents listed here.

COMPONENT ONE   **Suppress Inflammation-Autoimmunity**
a. Vitamin C, 2000 mg in morning and evening
b. Whole adrenal gland supplement. Follow the instructions on the label.
COMPONENT TWO   **Regenerate Tissues**
a. Colostrum, 500 mg daily or dehydroepiandrosterone (DHEA), 50 to 100 mg in the morning and evening
b. Polypeptide: Body Protection Compound (BPC-157) sublingual 100 to 200 mg three to five times a week
COMPONENT THREE   **Pain control**
a. Palmitoylethanolamide (PEA) with luteolin, 300 - 600 mg. Take one to three a day as needed for pain
b. Polypeptide-lysine, proline, valine (KPV) oral or nasal spray. Follow the instructions on the label.

NOTE: The above natural and herbal agents can be taken with other medications. All the above-listed medicinals can be obtained in health food stores or over the internet.

Step Nine: Prepare to Seek Medical Help

Compile all your medical records including MRIs and laboratory reports. Put all your records in an orderly file or three-ring binder. Take all your medical records with you when you attend a medical practitioner or pharmacy. Be prepared to show your records to physicians.

You have an uncommon severe, life shortening disease. Your medical practitioners will likely not know a lot about AA, so it will be up to you to put together a portfolio of your records, history, symptoms, and treatment plan to assist your doctor. If you simply go to a medical practitioner and say you have AA, the practitioner will likely tell you that your case is too complex, and he/she can't or won't help. If you just complain about your pain, chances are that your medical practitioner will just assume you are a drug seeker and refuse to treat you.

Handbook for Newly Diagnosed Cases of AA

Here is what must be in your portfolio to take to your medical practitioners:

A. Your MRIs and accompanying reports documenting that you have AA.

B. A list of the symptoms and complications that AA has produced. See Appendix.

C. Documents that validate the cause of your AA.

D. Take to your doctor a copy of the starting three-component medical protocol that is in the Appendix of this handbook.

E. Inform your medical practitioners as to the physical, medical, and nutritional measures that you have already started. Let your medical practitioner know you are studying the disease and are trying to help yourself. Your medical practitioner will likely be extremely busy and will appreciate education material about AA.

F. Common drugs for AA that a physician must prescribe include low dose naltrexone, ketorolac, methylprednisolone, or dexamethasone, and possibly opioids or other pain-relieving drugs.

G. The handbook "Clinical Diagnosis and Treatment of AA" and/or a copy of this handbook may be appreciated by your medical practitioners.

You will have to most likely rely on your local medical practitioners for help with prescription drugs as specialists in AA do not yet exist except in a few communities. You may have to search for a medical practitioner who will accept you. Avoid any medical practitioner who wants to give you an epidural injection, prolotherapy, surgery, or any other procedure until you are well stabilized on a three-component medical protocol with supporting nutrition and physical measures.

Step Ten: Start Spinal Fluid Flow Exercises

Exercises to enhance spinal fluid flow are a new concept in the care of AA. This author considers them to be essential.

<u>Facts About Spinal Fluid:</u> Spinal fluid is made in the brain, and it enters a enclosed flow or "pipe" system that carries the fluid around the brain, and then down the spinal canal. It turns around at the bottom (lumbar-sacral) area of the spine and is <u>pumped</u> upward to return to the brain and neck. Then it is <u>filtered</u> by lymph nodes and emptied into the general blood circulation to be excreted by one's kidneys. Spinal fluid has three major functions: (1) lubrication of the spinal cord and nerve roots, (2) carry nutrients, medications, and hormones, to the spinal cord and nerve roots, and (3) cleanse and wash away inflammation, toxins, and infectious agents.

Amazingly, spinal fluid is so precious to the proper function of the brain and spinal cord that new spinal fluid is made about every four to six hours. In other words, you have brand new spinal fluid three to four times a day.

<u>Problems For AA Patients</u>: AA is a result of inflammation and autoimmunity in the cauda equina nerve roots. Consequently, nerve roots form adhesions and clumps and may glue themselves to the inner wall (arachnoid) of the spinal canal covering. A mass is formed inside the spinal canal which is analogous to a boulder in a creek. Fluid flow is, therefore, diverted, backed up, and/or slowed down. Any obstruction, disruption, or diversion of spinal fluid flow may cause any or all the problems and symptoms listed here.

<u>Problems</u>	<u>Symptoms</u>
Poor Healing, Poor Response to Medication, Increased Pain, Leakage	Dizziness, Headache, Blurred Vision, Ear Ringing, Facial Pains

Handbook for Newly Diagnosed Cases of AA

We recommend exercises to keep spinal fluid rapidly moving to avoid problems and symptoms: Do one or more of the following exercises every day.

- ✓ Rock in a rocking chair
- ✓ Trampoline walking (rebounding)
- ✓ Deep breathe – hold for 5 seconds and slowly exhale with pursed lips

Summary

This handbook is primarily designed to help a person who has just received a diagnosis of AA. The ten steps provided are to help build a broad-based treatment program within sixty days. After sixty days you will undoubtedly want to undergo some testing for viral infection, inflammation activity, and hormone deficiencies. You should at that time try some ancillary treatments such as electromagnetic administration, hyperbaric oxygen, or stem cells.

Persons who have had AA for some time and are in a late stage of the disease will hopefully find this handbook helpful. New knowledge and therapeutic measures are being identified with regularity. This handbook has been written in mid-2023 with our best knowledge. Our bottom-line message is to get started without delay since AA deterioration is unpredictable and can be debilitating. Don't delay while searching or waiting for competent medical help, because your outcome may depend more on your personal efforts than what a medical practitioner can do for you.

Appendix

A. Symptom Criteria for the Diagnosis of AA

If a person has three or more of the following symptoms, a contrast lumbar-sacral MRI is warranted to see if AA may be the cause. If four or five symptoms are present, AA is almost certainly the cause.

1. Constant back pain with stabbing or shooting pains into the buttocks, hips, legs, or feet.
2. Pain is lessened by standing or reclining.
3. Burning or electrical shocks in feet.
4. Sensation of insects or water on the legs.
5. Difficulty starting, stopping, or holding urination.

B. Consequences and Complications of AA

AA has serious consequences and complications which may cause immense suffering, neurologic impairments, and shortened lifespan. This Table is presented to inform all concerned parties that AA is so serious that some therapeutic measures with risks may be warranted.

COMPLICATION	CONSEQUENCES
SPINAL FLUID FLOW OBSTRUCTION	➢ Headache ➢ Blurred vision ➢ Tinnitus (Ringing in ears) ➢ Mental impairments (memory, attention, reading, and mathematics)
SPINAL FLUID FLOW LEAKAGE	➢ Contraction of paraspinal muscles ➢ Tissue over lumbar spine indents or "caves in" ➢ Arms can't extend
SITTING/ STANDING ABILITY IMPAIRED	➢ Can't sit or stand in one position very long
INTRACTABLE PAIN SYNDROME	➢ Constant ("24/7") pain Cardiovascular, metabolic, and endocrine dysfunctions
NEUROPATHIC SYMPTOMS	➢ Burning feet ➢ Shooting pains into buttocks or legs ➢ Radiating type pain
IMPAIRED IMMUNITY	➢ Sepsis (infection) ➢ Premature death

LOSS OF BLADDER, BOWEL, AND SEXUAL FUNCTION	➢ Urgency, incontinence, hesitancy, or paralysis ➢ Bloating, abdominal pain, alternating constipation, and diarrhea ➢ Sex organs disabled, loss of libido
LEG AND FOOT PARALYSIS	➢ Weakness ➢ Inability to stand or walk ➢ Foot drop
BIZARRE NEUROLOGIC SYMPTOMS	➢ Sensation of water or insects on legs ➢ Burning of feet or buttocks ➢ Leg jerking, spasms, "restless legs"
DIETARY DYSFUNCTION	➢ Loss of appetite for proteins ➢ Excess sugar intake ➢ Malnutrition/weight loss ➢ Anorexia
HORMONAL DEFICIENCIES	➢ Cortisol ➢ Pregnenolone ➢ Dehydroepiandrosterone (DHEA) ➢ Testosterone

C. Stages and Categorizations of AA

Stage One – Mild

- Extremities: full range of motion, strength, extension
- No urinary or central symptoms*
- Normal ambulation
- Intermittent pain: non-opioid management is sufficient

Stage Two – Moderate

- Extremities: full range of motion, strength, extension
- Some urinary, gastrointestinal tract, and/or central symptoms*
- Normal ambulation
- Constant pain: non-opioid management is sufficient

Stage Three – Severe

- Extremities: some deficiency in range of motion, strength, extension
- Significant urinary, gastrointestinal tract, and/or central symptoms*
- Ambulates with assistance
- Severe, constant pain that requires daily opioids

Stage Four – Catastrophic

- Extremities: significant deficiency in range of motion, strength, extension
- Significant urinary, gastrointestinal tract, and/or central symptoms*
- Bed bound part of each day
- Ambulation requires assistance
- Severe, intractable pain that requires palliative care

Notes on Interpretation

*Central refers to headaches, and eye/ear/nasal symptoms such as blurred vision, tinnitus, vertigo, or nasal dripping.

*Ambulation assistance means cane, walker, wheelchair.

> MRI findings do not necessarily correlate with staging although the severe and catastrophic categories usually show one or more of these findings: dense scarring of nerve root clumps, multiple clumps, lower spinal canal distension ("empty sac"), peripheralization of nerve roots, calcification.

Note: Categories can overlap. Mild and moderate categories have the best potential for recovery.

D. Diagnostic Screening Test for Ehlers Danlos Syndromes (EDS)

Many people with AA do not know they have a genetic connective tissue disorder.

1. Has anyone in your family had Ehlers-Danlos Syndrome, Marfan syndrome, or a ruptured organ or aneurysm?

2. Have you developed a sudden, without warning or trauma, loss, or impairment of a neurologic function such as lifting, urination, flexing, or had a ruptured organ or aneurysm?

3. Have you had any teeth totally deteriorate or fall out?

4. Have you developed a sudden, constant pain in one spot on your body without warning or trauma?

5. Do you have any deformities or your hands or feet?

6. Can you now (or could you ever) place your hands flat on the floor without bending your knees?

7. Can you now (or could you ever) bend our thumb to touch your forearm?

8. As a child did you amuse your friends by contorting your body into strange shapes or could you do splits?

9. As a child or teenager did your shoulder or kneecap dislocate on more than one occasion?

10. Do you consider yourself double jointed?

11. Does your skin easily break, tear, crack, or bruise?

If you answered yes to four or more of these questions, you likely have a Ehlers-Danlos Syndrome or other genetic connective tissue disorder.

E. Diagnostic Screening Test for An Autoimmune Disorder

People with AA quite often are unaware that they have an autoimmune disorder. They often have multiple organ symptoms and dysfunctions prior to the development of AA, but don't consider AA part of their autoimmune disorder.

If you have five or more of the conditions listed here, you likely have an autoimmune disorder. It may be related to a silent infection such as Epstein Barr Virus (EBV), cytomegalovirus, or Lyme.

1. Arthritis
2. Burning mouth or feet
3. Carpal tunnel
4. Chiari conditions
5. Cold hands – Raynaud's
6. Dry eyes - Sjogren's
7. Dysautonomia (unstable blood pressure)
8. Fibromyalgia
9. Food-medicine sensitivities
10. Hashimoto's thyroiditis
11. Herniated/slipped discs
12. Herpes cold sores
13. Herpes genitalia
14. Spinal canal cysts (Tarlov's)
15. Irritable bowel
16. Mast cell activation

17. Migraine
18. Small fiber neuropathy
19. Psoriasis
20. Rheumatoid arthritis
21. Shingles
22. Spinal fluid leaks
23. Systemic lupus
24. Temporal mandibular joint (TMJ)
25. Urticaria (hives)

F. Start and Stop Rule for Pharmaceuticals

To effectively treat AA, one must sometimes try several therapeutic agents to find one that works. Follow the "start-stop" rule. Try a new pharmaceutical agent including natural and herbal agents for 15 days. If it relieves pain and provides more energy and sense of well-being, continue it. If not, stop it. If the therapeutic agent causes side effects at any time, stop it.

Every person who must take multiple pharmaceuticals should periodically ask "Is this agent still helping?" If you aren't sure, stop it. If you find out it was helping you, restart it.

Skip-Days Rule

The most popular and effective drugs for AA should not be taken every day unless absolutely necessary to get out of bed and function. This list includes ketorolac, methylprednisolone, dexamethasone, low dose naltrexone, polypeptides, colostrum, DHEA, nandrolone, human chorionic gonadotropin (HCG), PEA, gabapentin, prednisone, pure adrenal gland.

Here are some "skip-day" suggestions:

    a. Ketorolac, one to three days a week.
    b. Methylprednisolone, prednisone, or dexamethasone, one to three days a week.
    c. Hormones: DHEA, colostrum, human chorionic gonadotropin (HCG), pregnenolone, three to five days a week.

G. Physician's Starting Three Component Medical Protocol

<u>Component One (Suppression of Autoimmunity and Inflammation)</u>:

a. Palmitoylethanolamide (PEA) with luteolin (Mirica™, Glialia™, or other) 300 to 600 mg once or twice a day on three to five days a week.
b. Whole or pure adrenal gland supplement three to five days a week. Follow label instructions.
c. Ketorolac ten to thirty mg one or two times a week (oral, troche, injection) Option: diclofenac, twenty-five mg, twice or three times a day on three to five days a week.
d. Methylprednisolone oral two to four mg one or two times a week. (Option: ten mg by injection one to two times a month.)

Component Two (Regeneration of Tissue):

a. *BPC-157 polypeptide (Body Protective Compound) sublingual tablet, 100 mg. May combine with TB (Thymosin Beta) 500 mg. Take one to two dosages a day on three to five days a week.
b. Colostrum, 500 mg, or DHEA 50 mg, one to two dosages a day on three to five days a week.
c. KPV polypeptide (lysine, proline, valine) Oral or nasal spray on three to five days a week. Follow label instructions.

Component Three (Pain Control):

a. Continue any medication, including an opioid, that is providing pain relief.
b. If not on opioids, low dose naltrexone (LDN), one mg in AM and PM.
c. Any gamma amino butyric acid (GABA) surrogate: gabapentin, pregabalin (Lyrica®), diazepam (Valium®) alprazolam (Xanax®) topiramate (Topamax®) or other.

d. Sleep aid if necessary: amitriptyline, tryptophan or other.
  e. Pain flares: ketorolac ten to thirty mg and/or methylprednisolone ten to twenty mg by injection.
     Option: Six-Day Medrol® Dose Pak.

Notes:

1. Dosages and frequencies of all medications will almost always need to be changed over time.
2. Add ancillary treatments such as electromagnetic therapy or additional medications once this protocol is in place.
3. Specific dietary and physical measures are deemed essential in support of this protocol. They are provided in the Step Section of this handbook.
4. Unless necessary for pain control, we recommend that no medication be taken every day to avoid tolerance and side effects.

Glossary of Terms

<u>Adhesive Arachnoiditis:</u> An intraspinal canal inflammatory disorder in which there is a clump or mass of cauda equina nerve roots that are glued by adhesions to the arachnoid-dural covering of the spinal canal.

<u>Arachnoiditis-Non-Adhesive:</u> Inflammation of the arachnoid layer of the spinal canal covering (meninges) without any nerve roots adhered to it. This condition cannot specifically be identified by MRI. It is a clinical diagnosis based on signs, symptoms, and laboratory tests.

<u>Cauda Equina:</u> About two dozen nerve roots that emanate from the spinal cord at the level of the thoracic 12(T-12) or lumbar 1 (L-1) vertebrae and are suspended in spinal fluid.

<u>Clumping or Coalescence:</u> Multiple nerve roots have joined together due to inflammation and adhesion formation.

<u>Connective Tissue Disorder:</u> A genetic disease in which collagen in tissues deteriorates, weakens the tissues, and subsequently develops inflammation and pain in the tissues.

<u>Corticoid or Corticosteroid:</u> A pharmaceutical that is chemically related to cortisone.

<u>Epidural Injection:</u> An injection given in the space just above the spinal canal.

<u>Lumbar Spine:</u> A lower back section of the spine consisting of five vertebrae designated L1 through L5 with L1 being the topmost vertebrae.

<u>Meninges:</u> Spinal canal covering in the lumbar-sacral region that consists of an inside layer called arachnoid and an outer layer called the dura. The word "covering" is preferentially used in this handbook rather than meninges or theca to simplify understanding.

<u>Sacral Spine:</u> The lowest section of the spine which usually consists of three vertebrae. These vertebrae are designated S1, S2, and S3.

Spinal canal: Also known as the thecal sac. The spinal canal is a pipe like structure that carries the spinal fluid. The fluid is primarily produced in the brain and flows down the canal on one side and flows back up to the brain to be diverted into lymph nodes and the general blood supply.

Spinal Column: Refers to the entire spine including vertebrae, intervertebral discs, spinal canal, cord inside the canal, and cauda equina nerve roots.

Spinal Tap: A puncture of the spinal canal to either insert a substance into the canal or withdraw fluid from the canal.

References

1. Aldrete JA. History and evaluation of arachnoiditis: The evidence revealed. *Insurgentes Centro 51-A. Col San Rafael, Mexico* 2010; p3-14.
2. Aldrete JA. Suspecting and diagnosing arachnoiditis. *Pract Pain Mgt* 2006;16:74-87.
3. Aldrete JA. Arachnoiditis: the silent epidemic. *Future Med Publishers, Mexico* 2003
4. Anderson TL, Morris JM, Wald JT, et al. Imaging appearance of advanced chronic adhesive arachnoiditis: A retrospective review. *Am J Roentgenol* 2017;209:648-655.
5. Bilello J, Tennant F. Patterns of chronic inflammation in extensively treated patients with arachnoiditis and chronic intractable pain. *Postgrad Med* 2016;92:1-5.
6. Bjornevik, et al. Longitudinal analysis reveals high prevalence of Epstein-Barr virus associated with multiple sclerosis. Science 2022 Dol:10.1126/science.abj8222.
7. Burton C. Lumbosacral arachnoiditis. *Spine* 1978;3:24-30.

8. Castori M, Voermann NC. Neurological manifestations of "Ehlers-Danlos Syndromes. *Iran J of Neurol* 2014;13:190-208.
9. Delamarter RB Ross JS, Masaryk TS, et al. Diagnosis of lumbar arachnoiditis by magnetic resonance imaging. *Spine* 1990;15:304-310.
10. Eisenberg E, Goldman R, Schlag-Eisenberg D, et al. Adhesive arachnoiditis following lumbar epidural steroid injections: A report of two cases and review of literature. *J Pain Research* 2019;12:513-518.
11. Epstein NE. The risks of epidural and transforaminal steroid injections in the spine: commentary and a comprehensive review of the literature. *Surg Neurol* 2013;4 (supp2):574-593.
12. Harley JB, Chen X., Pujato M., et al. Transcription factors operate across disease loci, with EBNA2 implicated in autoimmunity. Nat Genet 2018;50:699-707
13. Harrow T. Epstein-Barr virus could be a cause of multiple autoimmune disorders. VA Research Currents April 18, 2018.
14. Henderson FC, Austin C, Benzel E, et al. Neurological and spinal manifestations of the Ehlers-Danlos Syndromes. *Amer J Men Gen* 2017;175C:195-211.

15. Horsley V. Chronic spinal meningitis: its differential diagnosis and surgical treatment. *Br J Med* 1909;1:513-517.
16. Jackson A, Isherwood I. Does degenerative disease of the lumbar spine cause arachnoiditis? A magnetic resonance study and review of the literature. *Brit J Radiology* 1994;67:840-847.
17. Jorgenson J, Hansen PH, Steenskoo V, et al. A clinical and radiological study of chronic lower spinal arachnoiditis. *Neuroradiology* 1975;9:139-144.
18. Kiefer R, Kreutzberg GW. Effects of dexamethasone on microglial activation in vitro. *J Neuroimmunology* 1991;34:99-108.
19. Kiguch et al. Chemokines and cytokines in neuroinflammation leading to neuropathic pain. Curr Opinion Pharmacol 2012;12:55-61.
20. Lei ZM, Rao CV. Neural actions of luteinizing hormone and human chorionic gonadotropin. *Seminar Reprod Med* 2001;19:103-109.
21. Loggia MI, Chunde DB, Oluwaseum A, et al. Evidence for brain glial activation in chronic pain patients. *Brain* 2015;138:604-615.
22. Parenti V, Huda F, Richardson PK, et al. Lumbar arachnoiditis: Does imaging associate with clinical features? *Clin Neurol Neurosurg* 2020;192:105717.

23. Quiles M, Marchiselo PJ, Tsairis P. Lumbar adhesive arachnoiditis: Etiologic and pathologic aspects. *Spine* 1978;3:45-50.
24. Rodriguez LJG, Sandoval SV, Rodriguez BD, et al. Paraplegia due to adhesive arachnoiditis: a case report. *Act Ortop Mex* 2009;23:232-236.
25. Sevesto S, Merli P, Ruggier M, et al. Ehlers-Danlos Syndrome and neurological features: a review. *Childs Neuro Syst* 2011;27:365-371.
26. Takahashi H, Suguro T, Okazima Y, et al. Inflammatory cytokines in the herniated disc of the lumbar spine. *Spine* 1996;21:218-224.
27. Takedo K. ,Sawamura S., Sekiyama H.,et al. Effect of methylprednisolone on neuropathic pain and spinal glial activation in rats. *Anesthesiology* 2004;100:1249-1257.
28. Tennant F. Human chorionic gonadotropin in pain treatment. *Prac Pain Manag* 2009;9:25-27.
29. Tennant FS Jr: The Glomerulonephritis of Infectious Mononucleosis. Texas Reports on Biology and Medicine 26:603-612, Feb 1969.
30. Thomas J. Arachnitis and Arachnoiditis. *Comprehensive Medical Dictionary. Philadelphia, J.B. Lippincott & Co.* 1873;p57.

31. Tsuda M. Microglia in the spinal cord and neuropathic pain. *J Diabetes Investig* 2016;7:17-26.
32. Whendon JM, Glassey D. Cerebrospinal fluid stasis and its clinical significance. *Altern Ther Health Med* 2009;15:54-60.
33. Zang Y, Chee A, Shi P, et al. Intervertebral disc cells produce interleukins found in patients with back pain. *Am J Phys Med* 2016;95:407-415.

Index

accident, 4, 25
adhesions, 4, 35, 54
arachnoiditis, 1, 54, 57, 60, 65
autoimmune, 26, 27, 47
burning, 39, 41, 42, 48
catastrophic, 44
collagen, 13
copper, 24
cytomegalovirus, 27, 48
dehydroepiandrosterone (DHEA), 29
deterioration, 12, 15, 37
diagnosis, 33, 39, 58
entraps, 6, 22
epidural, 4, 25, 33, 58
epsom, 23
epstein barr, 27, 48
flares, 53
function, 35, 46, 50
gabapentin, 50, 52
genetic, 4, 25, 45, 47, 55
goal, 12
herniated, 48

inflammation, 9, 10, 13, 14, 24, 27, 34, 35, 37, 54, 55, 57
inflammatory, 4, 6, 12, 18, 54
insects, 6, 39, 42
intervertebral discs, 56
ketorolac, 33, 50, 53
leakage, 18, 19
leaks, 49
lidocaine, 18, 19
lumbar, 2, 6, 34, 39, 41, 54, 55, 58, 59, 60
magnet, 23, 24
magnetic resonance imaging, 32
methylprednisolone, 33, 50, 53, 60
naltrexone, 33, 50, 52
nandrolone, 50
nerve root, 12, 22, 45
nerve roots, 4, 6, 22, 24, 34, 35, 45, 54, 56
pain, 24, 29, 35, 39, 52, 53, 57, 58, 60
palmitoylethanolamide, 29, 51
prednisone, 50

progression, 9
protein, 14
psoriasis, 27, 49
questions, 47
rocking, 36
scoliosis, 25
screening, 26
seepage, 18, 19
spinal fluid, 18, 19, 34, 35, 36, 54, 56
spinal tap, 26
spine, 18, 24, 34, 41, 55, 56, 58, 59, 60
spondylolisthesis, 26
surgery, 4, 26, 33
symptoms, 6, 9, 17, 31, 32, 35, 36, 39, 43, 44, 48, 54
systemic lupus erythematosus, 27
urination, 39, 46
vertebrae, 55, 56
vitamin, 29
water, 6, 22, 23, 39, 42
weight, 14, 42

OTHER BOOKS BY FOREST TENNANT

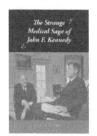

THE STRANGE MEDICAL SAGE OF JFK

ISBN:9781955934213
LOC:2023903440

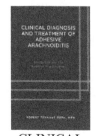

CLINICAL DIAGNOSIS AND TREATMENT OF ADHESIVE ARACHNOIDITIS
ISBN: 9781955934183
LOC: 2022907190

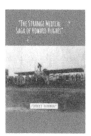

"THE STRANGE MEDICAL SAGA OF HOWARD HUGHES"
ISBN: 9781955934091
LOC: 2021912855

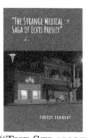

"THE STRANGE MEDICAL SAGA OF ELVIS PRESLEY"
ISBN: 9781955934008
LOC: 2021911718

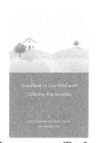

"HANDBOOK TO LIVE WELL WITH ADHESIVE ARACHNOIDITIS"

ISBN: 978195934060
LOC: 2021912718

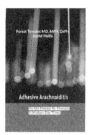

"ADHESIVE ARACHNOIDITIS: AN OLD DISEASE RE-EMERGES IN MODERN TIMES"

ISBN: 9781955934039
LOC: 2021912467

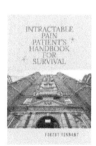

INTRACTABLE PAIN PATIENTS' HANDBOOK FOR SURVIVAL

ISBN: 9781955934121
LOC: 2021916464

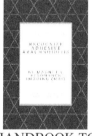

HANDBOOK TO RECOGNIZE ADHESIVE ARACHNOIDITIS BY MAGNETIC RESONANCE IMAGING (MRI)

ISBN: 9781955934152
LOC: 2021925161

Made in the USA
Las Vegas, NV
11 February 2025